I0814490

THE POCKET SELF-CARE

Published in 2026
by Gemini Gift Books
Part of Gemini Books Group

Based in Woodbridge and London

Marine House, Tide Mill Way,
Woodbridge, Suffolk IP12 1AP
United Kingdom

www.geminibooks.com

Part of the Gemini Pockets series

Cover image: Shutterstock/Kompor

ISBN 978-1-80247-354-4

A CIP catalogue record for this book is available from the British Library.

Disclaimer: This book is intended for general informational purposes only and should not be relied upon as recommending or promoting any specific practice or method of health treatments. It is not intended to diagnose, treat or prevent any illness or condition and is not a substitute for advice from a health care professional. You should consult your health practitioner before engaging in any of informational detailed in this book. You should not use the information in this book as a substitute for heath or other treatment prescribed by a professional practitioner. The publisher makes no representations or warranties with respect to the accuracy, completeness or currency of the contents of this work, and specifically disclaim, without limitation, any implied warranties of merchantability or fitness for a particular purpose and any injury, illness, damage, liability or loss incurred, directly or indirectly, from the use or application of any of the contents of this book. Furthermore, the publisher is not affiliated with and does not sponsor or endorse any methods of treatment or products referred in this book.

Manufacturer's EU Representative: Eurolink Compliance Limited, 25 Herbert Place, Dublin, D02 AY86, Republic of Ireland. admin@eurolink-europe.ie

Printed in China

10 9 8 7 6 5 4 3 2 1

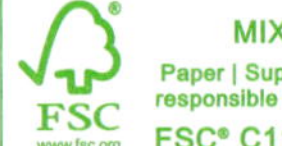

Picture Credits: 4, 7, 12, 48, 84, 102: Getty/Malte Mueller; 16: Shutterstock/Sviatlana Herasimenka; 17: Shutterstock/Yauheniya_Bandaruk; 21, 24, 27, 31, 32, 33, 34, 36, 41, 64, 80, 89, 91, 95, 105, 113, 122, 126, 127: Adobe Stock; 8, 9, 42, 43, 46, 47, 54, 62, 72, 73, 124, 125: Freepik

THE POCKET

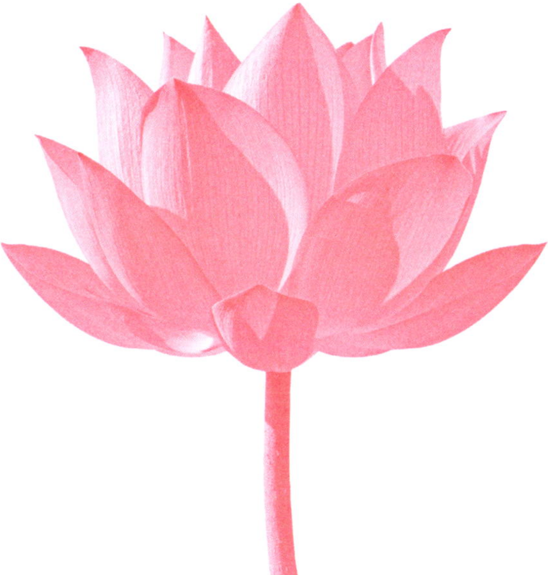

SELF-CARE

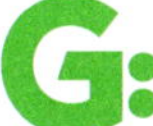

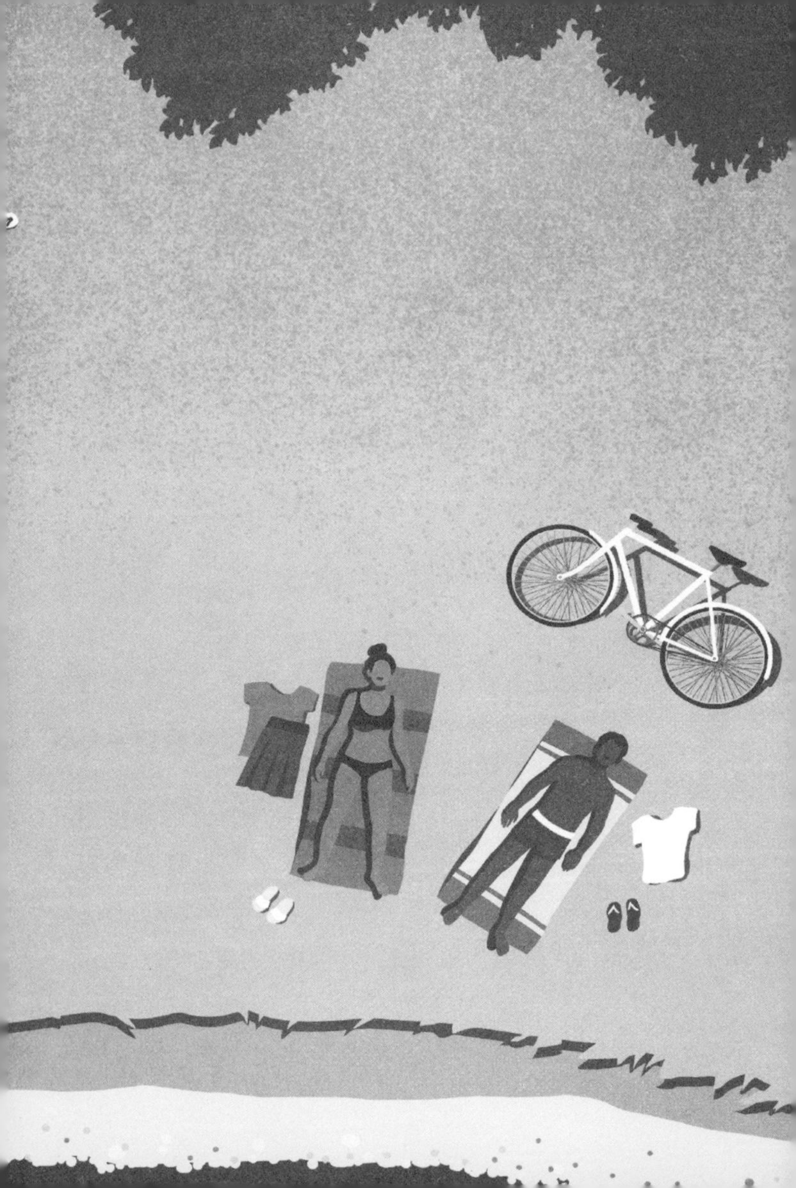

CONTENTS

Introduction

In our often-demanding modern world, self-care has become increasingly essential for our mental, physical and emotional wellbeing. So, whether you've recently recognized your need for more nurture or you're looking to improve an already existing self-care practice, this book offers you something special.

It's important to remember that self-care doesn't exist in isolation – it is linked to both community and environmental care. We all start from a different place, yet even the simplest self-care practice can help us all. You can read this book from cover to cover, or dip in and out as needed. Each section offers practical guidance that you can use straight away.

It's time to take care of you.

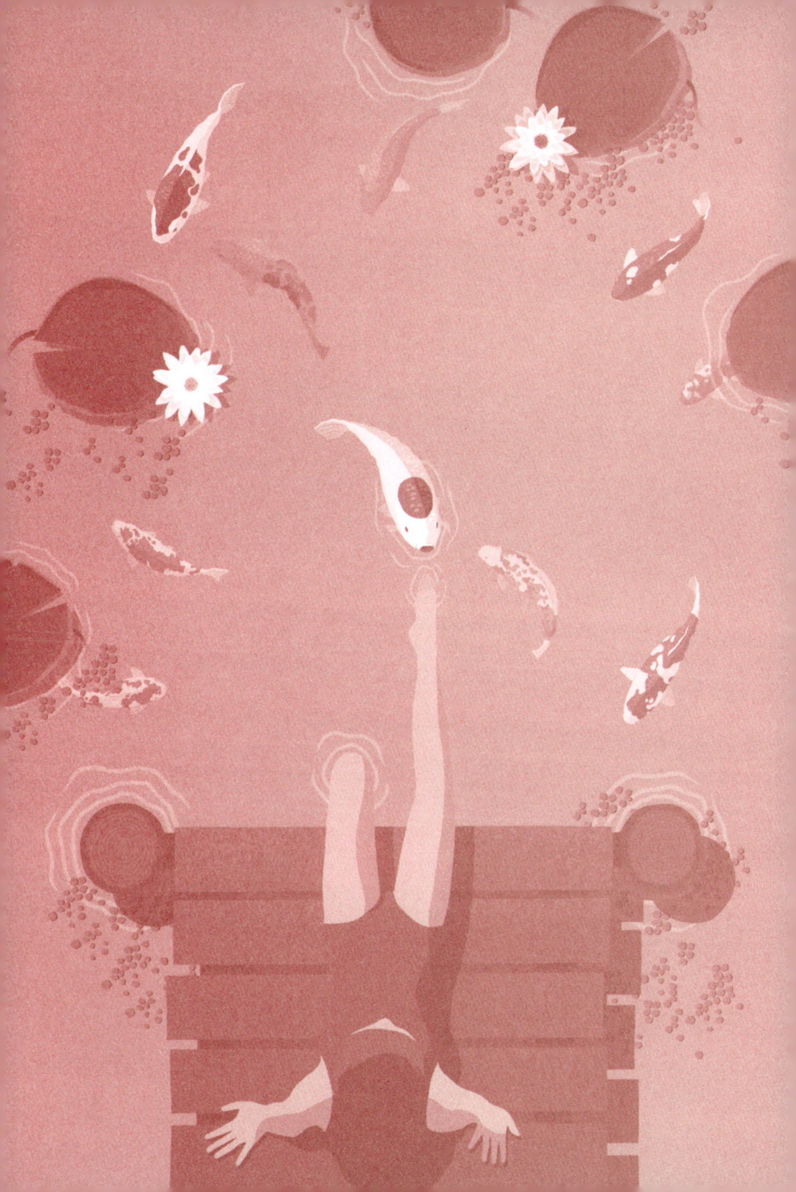

Self-care myths

Myth: Self-care is selfish

Truth: It allows you to show up for the people in your life more fully. Your wellbeing is connected to the wellbeing of others and the Earth.

Myth: Self-care is expensive

Truth: There are many low-cost ways to practise self-care, and some of the most important elements, such as setting boundaries, don't come with a financial price tag.

Myth: Self-care is all bubble baths and flowers

Truth: While a bubble bath with some rose petals can be a lovely way to nurture yourself, meaningful self-care often involves having tough conversations with yourself and others, as well as making difficult decisions.

Myth: Self-care takes lots of time

Truth: People often think that self-care takes hours to practise each day, but, in truth, many powerful methods can take just a few moments.

Myth: Self-care is for times of crisis

Truth: While self-care is important during the most challenging times of our lives, some of the most effective self-care is practised proactively during our moments of calm and clarity.

Myth: Self-care is an exciting new trend

Truth: Many of the practices in this book are inspired by traditions around the world, such as Japanese forest bathing or Danish principles of *hygge*. It is important to acknowledge that numerous cultures and indigenous peoples have practised self-care and community care for thousands of years, and continue to do so.

If you know your roots, it can be especially powerful to explore the self-care rituals woven through your lineage.

Start where you are

Here are our top five self-care starter tips:

1. Start where you are by beginning with the practices that feel the most easily accessible, achievable and – hopefully – fun!
2. Experiment and approach new practices with a curious mind. Take notice of how they make you feel and adapt them to suit your needs.
3. Keep a journal to record which practices help you the most, and be mindful of any patterns in how you feel.
4. Be gentle with yourself. Self-care isn't meant to be yet another item on your to-do list to worry or feel guilty about.
5. Practise methods that suit your energy levels, abilities and preferences. The suggestions in this book are simply starting points.

There is no one right way to practise self-care – what matters most is finding what resonates with you and fits into your life. It is different for everyone, and it is completely normal to seek further help, therapy or medication for particularly difficult situations.

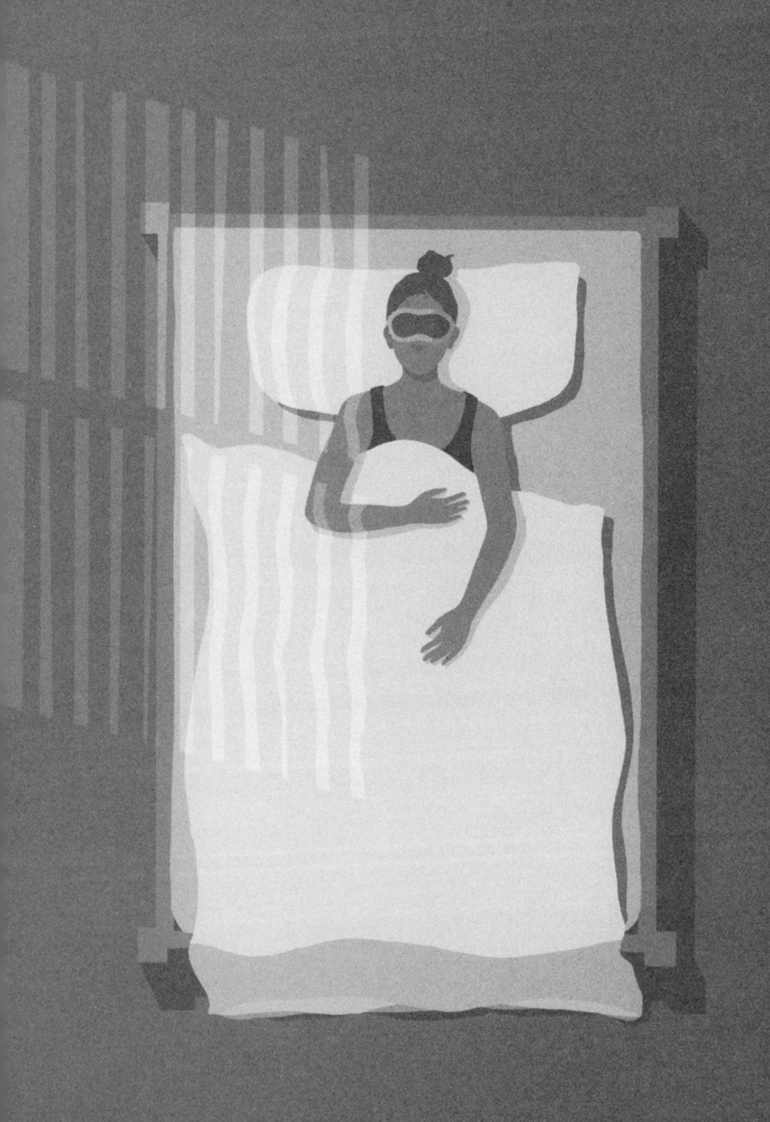

Chapter One

NOURISHING YOUR BODY

Your body deserves your care

Why relaxation matters

In today's busy world, it's easy to forget that relaxation is essential for both physical and emotional wellbeing – it should not be a luxury reserved only for the lucky few.

This is because when you are relaxed, your nervous system shifts from sympathetic (fight or flight) to parasympathetic (rest and digest), which is vital for your body to function properly.

It's not always easy to find the time to relax, so the key is to find small, simple ways to reduce stress. Hand-on-heart breathing is a great way to start and can be done daily.

Hand- on-heart breathing

Take a few deep breaths with your hands over your heart. Either close your eyes or soften your gaze, gently rub your hand against your heart in a circular motion.

Take five long, deep breaths and relax.

Sleep is vital

Sleep is an amazing healer – and it is essential for your health – yet it's often sacrificed for other things (or interrupted by small children!).

While the recommended amount of sleep for an adult is 7–9 hours, we often gloss over this underrated self-care practice. It is an act of self-care to prioritize sleep each night. Try setting a gentle alarm to remind yourself that it is time to wind down for sleep, and create a bedtime routine that soothes you.

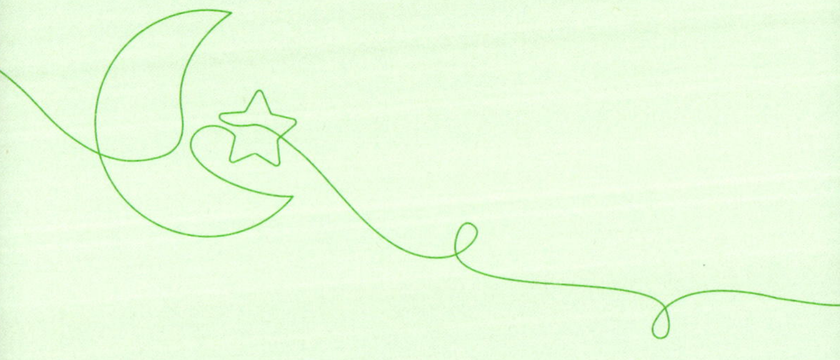

If you are a parent, it can be tempting to stay up late to have some time to yourself, but this can often leave you feeling more depleted. Try going to bed a little earlier, especially if you are woken regularly through the night.

Listen to your body and let it guide you in understanding how much sleep you need, rather than measuring yourself against others who may naturally require less rest. Every body is different, and some need more downtime than others.

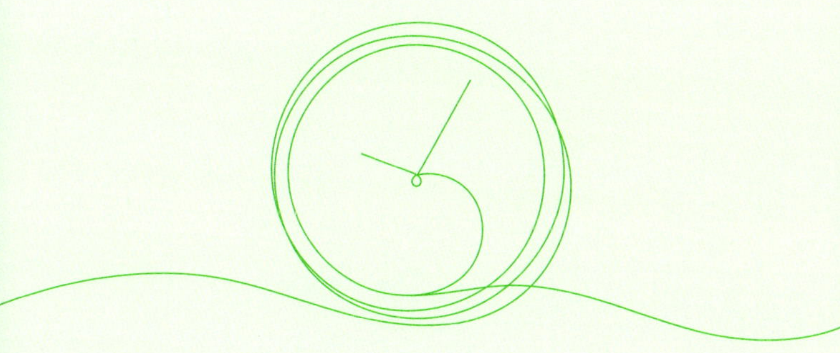

Create a sleep sanctuary

The environment you sleep in shapes the quality of your rest – use this checklist as part of your nightly self-care ritual:

- Put aside electronic devices (or switch them to "Do Not Disturb") and try not to use them for at least an hour before you sleep
- Wear blue light blocking glasses if you are exposed to screens in the evening
- Keep your room at a cool temperature (around 18°C)
- Keep the lighting low and gentle as you get ready for bed
- Use clean and fresh bedding if possible – it makes a difference!

- Wear comfortable, breathable clothing
- Choose calming, soft or neutral colours for your bedding and nightwear
- Keep your sleeping space clean and uncluttered
- Safely diffuse lavender essential oil or sip chamomile tea as you wind down
- Use blackout curtains or an eye mask to shield your eyes from any light
- Reduce unwanted background noise with earplugs

In many Scandinavian countries, it is common for couples to sleep with separate duvets, allowing each person to tailor their comfort to their own individual sleep preferences.

Bedtime routines

Consistent bedtime routines signal to your body and mind that it's time to move from day to night.

Choose gentle activities that help you unwind – like reading something light-hearted, listening to soothing music, doing some gentle stretching or writing in your journal. Some people find comfort in a nightly skincare routine or a warm shower or bath to wash away the day. The key is to discover out what feels right for you in this phase of life, and to treat it as a sacred part of your self-care.

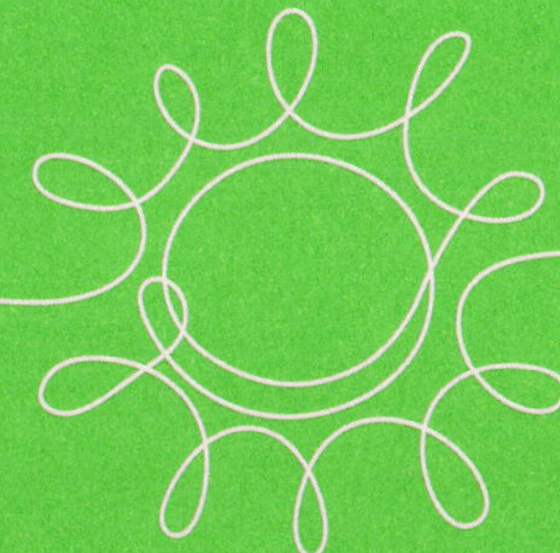

Try to maintain a regular sleep and wake time, even on weekends. On waking, try to spend time in natural lighting as soon as possible to help regulate your circadian rhythm (your body's internal clock).

Relaxation techniques

Simple techniques like belly breathing or body scanning can help to relax your body in preparation for sleep by activating your rest and digest system. Even 3–5 minutes of conscious relaxation can make a difference over time.

Belly breathing

Many of us never take a full deep breath unless we focus on doing so. To practise belly breathing, simply place your hands on your stomach and breathe in deeply through your nose. You will feel your hands rise and fall with each inhale and exhale.

Body scanning

This mindfulness practice involves slowly guiding awareness to each area of your body to pinpoint where you are holding tension and then actively releasing that tension. You can begin by breathing deeply through your belly and then slowly direct attention to your feet before gradually working your way through your body. Notice any tension and pain and breathe into them, allowing your body to acknowledge the sensation and relax.

You have permission to rest

In a world that often values productivity above all else, remember that rest is not lazy or a reward for hard work – it's necessary for all humans to be healthy. Your inherent worth is not measured by how active you are each day – or how hard you work. This book is your permission slip to slow down whenever you can – to nap, to doze, to daydream.

When you do rest, notice any guilt or other uncomfortable feelings that arise, and gently remind yourself that restoration is vital for all of life. Some people find resting extremely challenging – remember to be compassionate with yourself and take each day at a time.

"No need to hurry. No need to sparkle. No need to be anyone but oneself."

Virginia Woolf, *A Room of One's Own*

Connect to your body

Connecting with your body means nurturing a kind and loving relationship with yourself. For many, this can be complex – shaped by a range of experiences – so approach the process with gentleness, and don't hesitate to seek support if you need it.

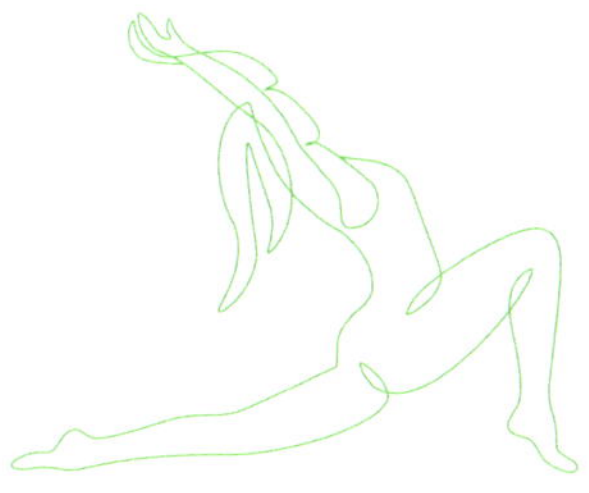

Yoga, Tai Chi, Qigong, Pilates, dance, breathwork, nature walks, body scan meditations, strength training, stretching, swimming, self-massage, mindful eating, cold/warm water therapy and even gardening can create a stronger awareness of your body.

Come back to the breath

Bringing your attention to your breath during the day is one of the simplest ways to connect to your body - and it is free. We tend to breathe through our mouths when we are in fight or flight mode, so consciously breathing through the nose can help us relax.

Deepen your breath for 5–10 slow inhales and exhales to activate your parasympathetic nervous system. Try extending your exhale to be longer than your exhale.

Box Breathing

1. Inhale slowly through your nose for a count of four.

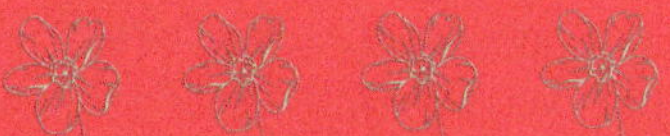

2. Hold your breath for a count of four.

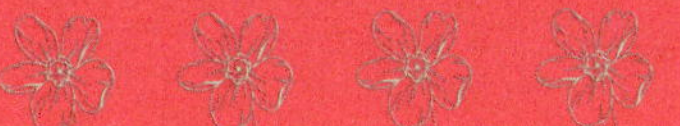

3. Exhale slowly through your mouth for a count of four.

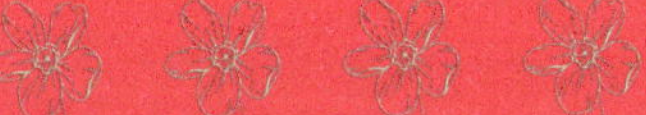

4. Hold your breath for a count of four.

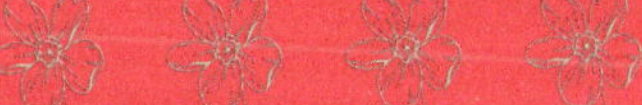

5. Repeat five times.

Walk in nature

Mindful walking involves consciously tuning into your surroundings as you walk – whether that's along a country path or in your local park. If walking isn't possible, you can engage in this practice by simply sitting somewhere quiet, perhaps on a bench or on your doorstep.

As you walk, notice the sensation of your feet touching the ground. Bring awareness to your breath, and slowly tap into the essence of the nature around you – the drifting clouds, the call of birds, the rustle of trees, the whisper of the wind. Acknowledge each element as it passes you, recognizing that you, too, are a part of nature.

Forest bathing is a self-care practice developed in Japan. It invites you to slowly and mindfully walk through woodland, fully immersing yourself in the sights, sounds and scents of the natural world.

Connect to the Earth

This simple barefoot grounding and breathing practice offers an easy way to connect with the natural world and anchor yourself in the present moment.

1. Set a timer with a gentle alarm for 5–10 minutes.
2. Either standing, sitting or lying down, press your feet (or body) firmly into the ground – ideally on a natural surface such as grass, sand or even mud.
3. Feel how the Earth supports you, then, if standing, sway from side to side a few times.

4. Name five things you can see, four things you can touch, three things you can hear, two things you can smell and one thing you can taste.
5. Breathe in slowly through your nose for a count of four, hold for a second or two, then exhale through your nose for a count of six.

Swimming in a lake or the ocean - or even paddling in a stream - can be a beautiful way to connect with nature. So too can feeling the sun on your face in the early morning, or pausing to watch the colours of the sunset in the evening.

Move your body

Including movement in your day is an important part of self-care. It becomes energizing when you discover a form of exercise that brings you joy, rather than feeling like a chore.

It can be as simple as dancing freestyle to your favourite music as you cook, as adventurous as open-water swimming in natural rivers, or as simple as practising a few gentle yoga poses while lying on your bed. The most important thing is to find a movement practice that is sustainable and enjoyable for you.

Different bodies need different kinds of movement – high-intensity exercise might feel great to one person but not to another. The key is to honour your body by finding something that feels good.

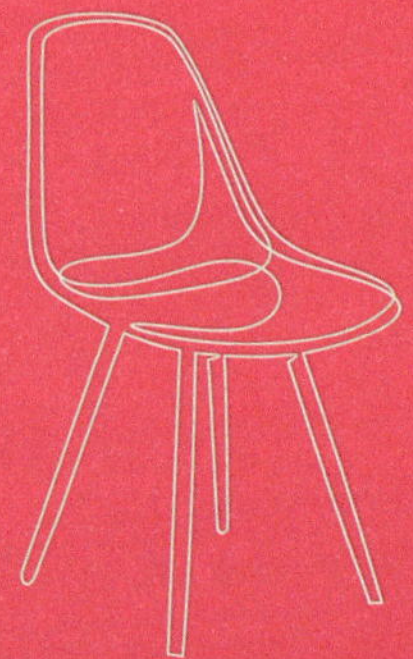

Chair yoga

Chair yoga can be practised any time throughout the day – even at work – and can help you feel stronger, more flexible and more grounded.

Sit upright in a chair with your hands on your knees. Take three deep breaths before you begin.

1. Gently tilt your right ear toward your right shoulder. Hold for 5 seconds, then repeat on the left.
2. Circle your shoulders backward three times, then forward three times.
3. Place your right hand on your left knee and your left hand behind the chair. Gently twist left and look over your shoulder. Hold for 5 seconds, then repeat on the other side.
4. Lift your right foot a few inches from the ground and circle your ankle five times clockwise, and then again anticlockwise. Repeat with your left foot.
5. With your feet flat on the floor, slowly bend forward and let your arms hang down to the ground. Hold for 5 seconds then slowly rise back up.
6. Raise your right arm overhead and gently lean to the left. Hold for 5 seconds, then repeat on the other side.
7. Take three deep, calming breaths before continuing your day.

Nourishing nutrition

Choosing foods that support your body is an important element of self-care. Instead of focusing on restricting so-called "bad" foods, try to shift your attention towards adding more nourishing options - such as including extra green vegetables in your meals, or swapping a chocolate bar for a handful of nuts or seeds. Begin to see your relationship with food, and with your digestion, as an ongoing journey of exploration. Take time to learn about your gut health, experiment with what feels good for you, and seek professional guidance if needed.

A lovely way to rediscover joy in eating and cooking is by reconnecting with recipes from your heritage or by exploring how different cultures celebrate food. With so many vibrant flavours and dishes to choose from, the process can be both exciting and enriching. Plus, cooking and sharing a meal with friends or family can be a wonderful experience!

"The greatest wealth is health."

Roman poet Virgil (70BC–198BC)

Mindful eating

Rooted in Buddhism, mindful eating invites us to slow down and be fully present as we focus on the sensory experience of each mouthful. It is an ancient practice that encourages awareness of the tastes, textures, smells and even sounds of food as we eat, fostering a deeper connection between mind and body.

In today's fast-paced world, where eating is often rushed or done while distracted, mindful eating offers a valuable way to reconnect with both the act of eating and the body's natural rhythms. Whether applied to a single meal or integrated into daily life, it encourages self-awareness, gratitude and balance – principles that not only support physical health but also contribute to overall mental and emotional wellbeing.

Top tips for conscious eating

- Take small bites and chew each mouthful thoroughly
- Notice the colours, scents and textures of your food
- Rest your cutlery between each bite to tune into your hunger signals
- Eat without distractions, including screens
- Use your favourite kitchenware items, such as your favourite plate or glass
- Decorate your tabletop with flowers or candles (or both!)

The environment in which you eat, the people you eat with and how much you enjoy your food all makes a difference.

Budget-friendly food

Eating consciously and nutritiously can be expensive, but there are ways to build a nourishing diet with simple, affordable foods that you can easily cook at home.

Lentils, beans, eggs, whole grains and seasonable vegetables are great options – if they are suitable for your digestive system. Buying in bulk can help reduce costs, and, if possible, try growing your own herbs, salads or vegetables at home. Even a windowsill can provide enough space to grow spring onions or lettuce.

Another useful tip is to save beef or chicken bones to make a nourishing stock, which can be sipped as a broth or used as a base for soups and other homemade dishes.

Cooking from scratch using whole ingredients is a great way to make meals that yield multiple portions and ultimately save money.

Keep an eye on reduced-to-clear sections in supermarkets for items you can cook or freeze right away. And finally, batch cooking is another smart way to save money, allowing you to stretch meals like stews and curries over several days.

Gentle self-care during illness

Though often unwelcome, illness can offer an invitation to practise deeper self-care and compassion. During these often challenging times, even the simplest acts of self-care can take on greater meaning.

If you're unwell, allow this time to become a moment of self-enquiry. Reflect on what is truly supporting you – and what isn't any longer. Try this journalling prompt: Does your body have a message for you that you have been too busy to hear?

For those with chronic conditions, illness may require a different, more adaptable approach. While some people benefit from strong support systems and paid time off, many face long-term illness without the resources or care they need. If this is your reality, be gentle with yourself and avoid comparing your journey to those of others.

Including community care within your self-care practice is a powerful reminder that we are all interconnected. When we care for one another, we create spaces where everyone has a chance to heal and thrive.

Hydration and energy

Water is essential for our wellbeing, making proper hydration a key part of self-care. It supports everything from digestion and skin health to energy levels, mood and even brain function.

When we're well hydrated, we tend to feel more balanced – both physically and emotionally. Sipping water regularly is a gentle way of checking in with ourselves, a reminder to slow down and care for our bodies. Whether it's starting the day with a glass of water, keeping a bottle nearby while working or enjoying herbal teas in the evening, staying hydrated is one of the easiest ways to support our overall wellbeing.

Top tips to stay hydrated

- Carry a reusable water bottle when you're on the go
- Drink little and often – before you get too thirsty
- Set reminders on your phone to encourage you to drink at regular times
- Keep a water jug near you on a table or desk
- Try adding some sliced cucumber, lemon or even fruit to your water for extra hydration
- Eat foods with a high water content, such as salads and watermelon

Always remember that everyone's needs are different. Your activity levels, the climate you live in and your body's unique requirements all play a part.

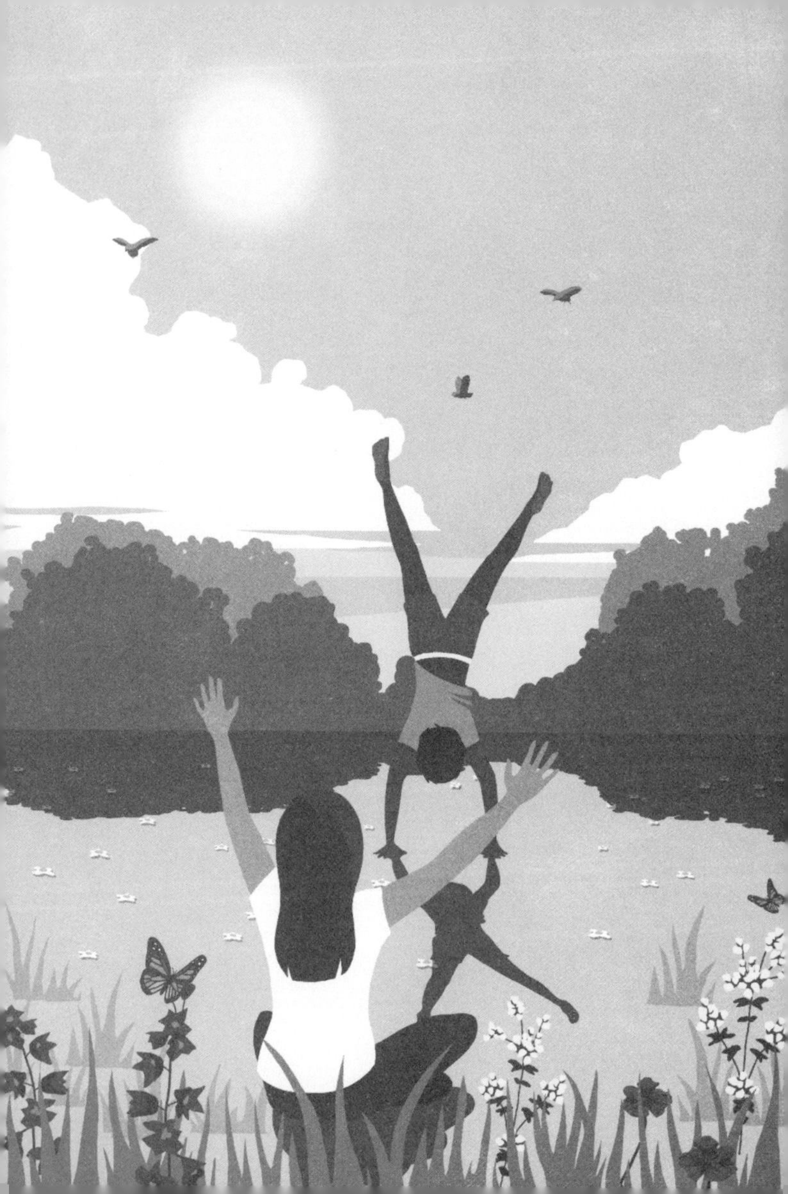

Chapter Two

TENDING TO YOUR HEART AND MIND

Your emotional wellbeing matters

What is emotional self-care?

Caring for your emotions can mean:

- ♥ Acknowledging your feelings in a non-judgemental way
- ♥ Fully feeling all emotions that arise in you
- ♥ Finding healthy ways to express, process and integrate your emotional responses

When you learn to listen to and nurture your emotions, you build resilience to stress and, just as importantly, develop the capacity for deeper connections with yourself and others.

This chapter explores gentle ways to tune in and begin understanding the messages that your emotions are trying to share.

Emotional awareness

One of the first steps toward emotional awareness is noticing where emotions arise in your body. Take a moment now to tune in.

Is there a flutter of excitement in your stomach? A heavy sadness sitting on your chest? Perhaps a mixture of both – or something else entirely. Once you have located an emotion, try naming it. Some people find this helpful, while others prefer to simply sit with the sensation, allowing to exist without resisting or labelling.

What feels right for you? Both approaches – naming the emotion or resting in silent awareness – can strengthen your ability to be with all feelings and emotions.

Notice any ways you might be avoiding your emotions. Perhaps you reach for your phone to scroll or turn to food for comfort. If so, meet yourself with compassion. Stay away from judgement, and simply do your best to to stay present with whatever is arising. If it feels overwhelming, know that it's okay to seek support.

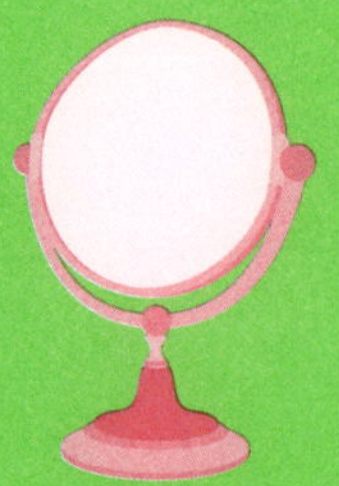

Self-forgiveness mirror ritual

One of the most truly challenging aspects of self-care is forgiveness – especially when it comes to ourselves. This simple yet powerful ritual invites you to practise self-forgiveness using your own reflection and the strength of your voice.

Don't underestimate the healing that can come from speaking kindly to yourself. Try this practice when you feel ready to release an emotional burden and move forward with greater compassion.

1. Look into a mirror and smile kindly at your reflection.
2. Take a few deep breaths then speak out loud: "I have been really hard on myself about [name the situation], but I acknowledge that I was doing the best I could with the tools I had. I now understand why I acted, felt and thought this way."
3. Place your hand on your heart and say: "I release this [guilt, shame or regret]. I choose to forgive myself and everyone else involved. I am worthy of forgiveness."
4. Look into your eyes and say: "Even though I cannot change the past, I can choose peace moving forward. I fully release this emotional burden and welcome a new reality."
5. Smile lovingly at yourself for a few moments, perhaps hug yourself as well, and continue with your day. Do this as many times as you need until the emotional burden is released.

Clearing energy

There are many ways to clear dense or lingering energy after a ritual like this. Some people choose to burn sage or other cleansing herbs, while others prefer sound – using tuning forks, bells or singing bowls. Even something as simple as clapping your hands for a few moments can help shift the energy.

"What lies behind us and what lies before us are tiny matters compared to what lies within us."

Ralph Waldo Emerson, *Essays*

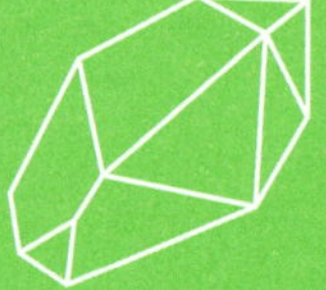

The best crystals for emotional self-care

Many people find comfort in working with crystals as part of their self-care journey. Crystals are believed to carry unique vibrational frequencies that can subtly interact with the body's energy field, offering support for emotional balance and healing. The following crystals are commonly used to support emotional wellbeing:

Rose quartz

(self-love)

This beautiful pink stone is associated with unconditional love and self-compassion

Amethyst

(soothing grief)

This crystal is known for its calming energy and is thought to bring comfort during challenging times

Carnelian

(self-confidence)

This bright orange-red stone is linked with courage and personal power; it is believed to boost self-belief and confidence

Black tourmaline

(emotional protection)

This grounding crystal helps with deflecting negativity and setting boundaries

Moonstone

(emotional intuition)

This particularly gentle crystal helps connect with feminine energy and intuition

Rhodonite

(healing heartache)

This pink and black stone is brilliant for healing after difficult relationships and for releasing emotional pain

Citrine

(abundance)

This bright yellow stone helps to encourage a positive outlook that can lift heavy feelings and inspire joy

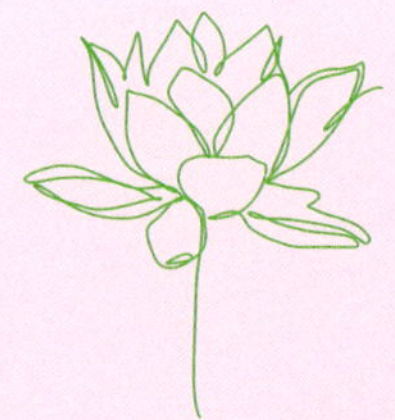

A self-love meditation

Meditation is a profound self-care practice that offers precious moments of stillness when your nervous system can rest and you can reconnect with yourself.

A short, grounding practice can help create space between thoughts, soften tension in the body and bring you back to the present. On the following page is a simple meditation you can return to whenever you need a pause, a reset or a gentle reminder to come home to yourself.

1. Sit in a comfortable position and take some deep breaths. Allow your body to relax.
2. Guide attention to your heart and imagine a beautiful golden light glowing in the centre of your chest.
3. Embrace the memory of a time when love filled you completely – feel it viscerally, then allow that warmth to spread through your body.
4. As this feeling flows through you, silently say: "I am love."
5. Rest for a few minutes to soak in the energy of love. When you're ready, open your eyes and continue with your day. Carry this reminder within you: You don't need to earn love – you are love itself.

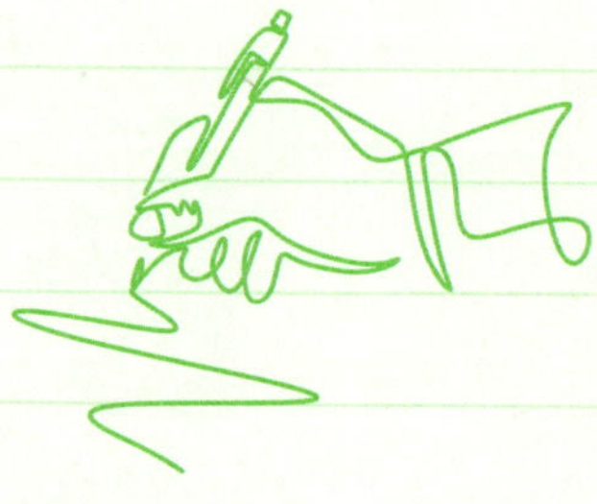

Did you know that even 5 minutes of free writing can help you process and move through your emotions?

Our most dominant thoughts can have a powerful impact on how we feel, and writing them down can bring those thoughts into our awareness, allowing us to release what no longer serves us.

Set a timer and write whatever comes crosses your mind, without judgement. No one else needs to read your words, and if it feels right to you, you can safely burn or tear up the paper when you're done.

You can write whenever you find a moment, though some people prefer to journal first thing in the morning or just before bed. If you're short on time, try jotting down bullet points on your phone or recording a voice memo. If writing isn't your thing, you might choose to sketch or use colour as a way to express what you're feeling.

Develop self-compassion

Self-compassion is the ability to be loving, kind and mindful to yourself when you experience difficult feelings or make mistakes. This compassion helps to create a sense of safety within, which is an essential part of self-care.

Developing self-compassion often requires consistency – especially if you tend to avoid your feelings or are highly self-critical. It can be easy to overlook the subtle ways we judge ourselves.

When difficult emotions arise, try to acknowledge them with kindness; if you catch yourself being self-critical, try to pause, take notice and gently bring your awareness back to compassion.

For example, if you see a photo of yourself that you don't like and catch yourself thinking something unkind about your appearance – pause and notice. Then, gently choose compassion instead. With time and practice, this kinder way of responding can begin to feel more natural.

These pauses are essential in self-compassion practice – they give you the space to truly feel the kindness you are offering yourself.

Simple self-compassion practice

Imagine taking care of others

If your inner critic is loud, try imagining how you would speak to a small child or a close friend who is experiencing a similar challenge. Notice how naturally compassion flows when someone else is vulnerable. Now, practise focusing that same tender, nurturing energy inward – offering it to yourself with the same care and kindness.

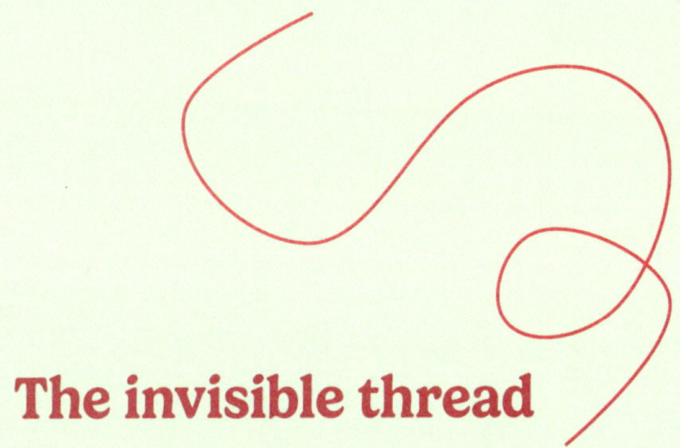

The invisible thread

In difficult moments, it can be comforting to remember that, all around the world, countless others are facing struggles similar to your own. Connecting with this sense of shared humanity is a powerful reminder that life as a human being means experiencing a wide spectrum of emotions – and that we are all far more connected than we often realize.

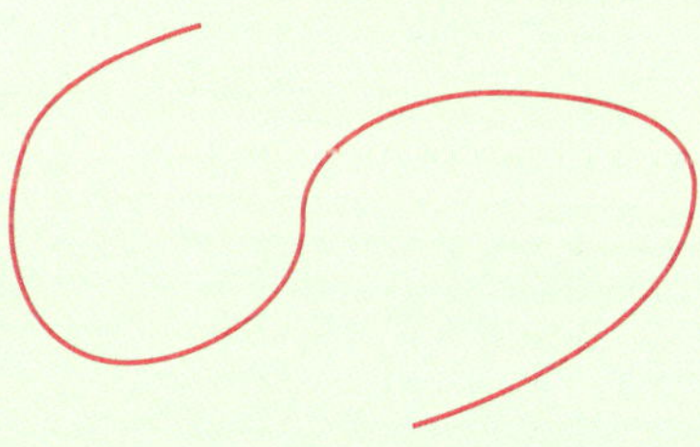

Transform your self-talk

Your inner voice – the way you speak to yourself – has a significant influence on your experience of life and how you show up in the world. Try to notice when your self-talk becomes dismissive or overly critical. For many people, this inner dialogue can be subtle, so it helps to pay close attention.

Begin by gently shifting the language you use with yourself, here are some examples:

"I always make mistakes"

Replace with: "I made a mistake, and that's okay – everyone does."

"I'll never manage that"

Replace with: "I'm finding this really hard right now."

"Financial opportunities never work out for me"

Replace with: "I'm telling myself a story about money that focuses only on disappointments. I have fears about money, and I am open to new, more supportive possibilities."

These small adjustments may seem simple, but over time, they can help you develop a more patient and compassionate relationship with yourself.

Personal affirmations

Personal affirmations are empowering phrases that can help shift negative self-talk over time. Repeating them is believed to strengthen positive neural pathways in the brain, gradually rewiring the way you think and feel about yourself.

At first, positive affirmations might feel uncomfortable – especially if you have held opposing beliefs for many years. If you notice resistance, gently acknowledge it and meet it with self-compassion. Remind yourself of this deeper truth: You are enough, you are worthy of good things and you deserve care – from yourself and from others.

Try speaking affirmations aloud while looking in the mirror, writing them in your journal or placing them somewhere visible throughout the day – like on your phone background or a sticky note placed on the fridge. These small moments of reinforcement can make a meaningful difference.

On the next page, you'll find a collection of affirmations to speak aloud – let their words settle into your heart and mind.

I am enough
I trust myself
I am safe
I choose peace
I am growing
I deserve rest
I am worthy of love
I believe in myself
I let go of fear

I am calm
I am resilient
I welcome joy
I honour my needs
I am kind to myself
I am doing my best
I embrace change
I radiate love
I am grounded
I deserve happiness
I am strong

Managing anxiety

Anxiety is one of the most common mental health challenges. It arises when the body's natural alert system becomes overactive, keeping you in a hightened state of worry or tension. While it's normal to feel anxious from time to time, chronic anxiety can be overwhelming and may require extra support to manage.

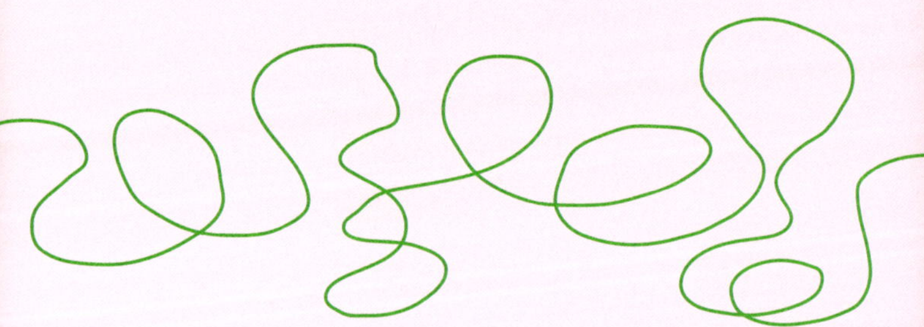

Sometimes, anxiety is a completely appropriate response to a difficult situation. It may be your body's way of alerting you to something that needs attention – perhaps a relationship, job or environment that is no longer supporting your wellbeing. In these cases, anxiety might be signalling the need to make an uncomfortable or difficult decision in order to feel safe again.

Restoring balance

Managing anxiety often means finding gentle practices that help you, as an individual, return to a sense of balance. This can look different for everyone. Some people find relief through movement, while others feel more at ease through creativity – such as writing, painting or playing music. For some, healing appears through sound, colour, crystal work or other holistic practices.

Holding space

While managing symptoms is an important part of self-care, understanding the root causes of anxiety can lead to deeper, more lasting change. This often involves nurturing the body, mind and spirit – and for many, working with trusted professionals can be a valuable part of the journey.

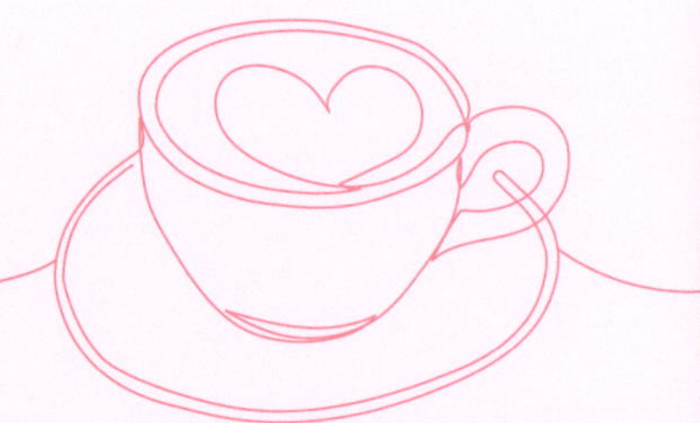

Build an emotional self-care kit

Creating an emotional self-care kit is a personal and empowering way of keeping sources of comfort close by. Here are some things you could include:

- A crystal – to hold or to wear as jewellery
- Your favourite essential oils – such as lavender, ylang ylang or rose
- Photographs of loved ones or special moments
- Comfy clothes that you love to wear
- A journal and a favourite pen
- Herbal teas – such as chamomile or mint
- A playlist with different themes for different emotions
- A book of spiritual wisdom or affirmations
- A stress ball, fidget toy or any sensory object
- A list of the most supportive people in your life – and their phone numbers

A little piece of magic

Every item in your emotional self-care kit will carry a small kind of magic – not because of what it is, but because of how it makes you feel. A soft hoodie that wraps you in warmth, a scent that instantly calms your breath or a photo that reminds you you're not alone. These are not luxuries; they are lifelines. Small, personal rituals that offer comfort when the world feels too loud or your heart feels too heavy.

Your kit isn't meant to "fix" you – it's there to hold space for you. To offer a gentle pause. A moment to remember that you are safe, supported and worthy of care.

There's power in preparing for your harder moments with softness. In choosing tools that honour your emotional landscape. In doing so, you remind yourself: I can meet myself where I am. And that's enough.

“I am not afraid of storms, for I am learning how to sail my ship.”

Louisa May Alcott, *Little Women* (1868–1869)

Chapter Three

CREATING NURTURING ENVIRONMENTS

Your surroundings shape your wellbeing in powerful ways

Environments matter

An often-overlooked aspect of self-care is the impact of the spaces we inhabit each day. This chapter invites you to reflect on your surroundings and consider how they support – or challenge – your wellbeing. Tending to your environment can be a meaningful and empowering act of self-care.

Home environments to assess:

- Bedroom
- Bathroom
- Home office or workspace/desk
- Kitchen/dining areas
- Living room
- Storage areas
- Car (if you have one)

For each environment, ask yourself:

1. How does this space make me feel when I enter it?

2. Which items support my well being and which ones evoke overwhelming emotions?

3. What is one small change that could make this environment more nurturing?

Making mindful improvements

Once you've assessed your home environments, you can begin to make some simple changes.

Remember:

- Designating small areas just for you can be a great start
- Removing clutter is more impactful than buying new things
- Houseplants, natural materials and images of nature can add a sense of calm

Top tips for decluttering

- Treat decluttering as a gentle way to reset rather than as a stressful chore
- Declutter or rearrange one small area (or just remove a few items) at a time (you can make this a game by choosing a specific item to clear first, such as gathering all red items, or putting away all your socks)
- Schedule decluttering time regularly
- Designate a specific home for everything you decide to keep
- Create separate keep, donate and sell piles
- If you are unsure about getting rid of something, put it aside and consider it again in a few months
- Declutter with a friend or family or listen to music, a podcast or an audiobook to make the process less stressful

Creating a meditation space

Designating a space for mediation can be a great way to encourage moments of stillness and inner connection. All you need is a quiet spot where you won't be disturbed, something comfortable to sit or lie down on, and – if it feels supportive – a few calming touches like candles, incense or soft lighting.

Top tips for meditation practice

- Wear loose, comfortable clothing
- Start with just a few minutes at a time and increase the time with each practice
- Try to meditate at the same time each day
- Take it easy and don't worry about doing it in a specific way – every way is the "right" way
- Use a meditation app or a guided video if you need support

Meditation helps you cultivate clarity, focus and insight by developing the ability to witness your thoughts rather than identify with them.

A bathing ritual for inner peace

Water has been a source for healing, cleansing and renewal across cultures for thousands of years. Try this simple evening bath ritual to soothe your body and calm your mind before bed.

1. Tidy your bathroom, dim the lights, safely light a candle and run the water for the bath.
2. Add a handful of Epsom salts and a few drops of your favourite essential oil mixed with some coconut oil.

3. Take a deep breath and speak your intention for inner peace.
4. Step in the bath, noticing the sensation of warm water on your skin and the scent of the oils. Take long slow breaths, and relax.
5. When you're ready, drain the water and visualize any stress flowing away. Wrap yourself in a soft towel before changing into comfortable nightwear and heading to bed.

Tip: Choose candles and nightwear in calming and peaceful colours, such as blue and white.

Creating a clear workspace

Whether you're working from an office or your kitchen table, your environment plays a big role in shaping your productivity and creativity.

A thoughtfully set-up environment, no matter how simple, helps signal to your brain that it's time to concentrate, create or even rest between tasks. Small details like natural light, calming colours, a tidy surface or even a favourite mug can all contribute to how motivated and grounded you feel throughout the day.

Creating a space that works with you – not against you – is one of the simplest ways to care for yourself while getting things done.

Top tips for a comfortable workspace

- Clear the clutter and add an inspiring object (or a few!) to to your workspace
- Ensure that your chair is in a comfortable position – or try a standing desk
- Place your feet flat on the floor
- Adjust your screen to eye level and regularly take breaks from looking at the screen – ideally, look out of a window to absorb some nature
- Keep a notepad and pen nearby – write down your tasks to keep organized lists of completed and pending tasks

Digital wellness quiz

Answer **YES** or **NO** to each question:

1. When I scroll through social media, I usually feel inspired.
2. I allocate certain times of day that are completely screen-free.
3. I regularly unfollow or mute social media accounts that affect me negatively.
4. At least one space in my home is a phone-free zone.
5. I take regular breaks from tech and social media.

6. I have daily limits on my devices for social media apps.
7. I clear unimportant notifications.
8. I choose when and how I engage with tech.
9. My online profiles reflect who I am and what matters to me.
10. I'm in charge of my tech use – not the other way around.

Your results:

8–10 YES answers:

You have strong self-awareness around your use of technology, and you're using digital tools in ways that support your energy and creativity – keep it up!

4–7 YES answers:

You're making good, thoughtful choices, but there's a little room for improvement. What is one small change you could make that might have the biggest impact right now? Perhaps a tech-free morning each week?

0–3 YES answers:

No judgement! Managing our digital lives is becoming more and more challenging. Take a moment to reflect on some small, sustainable small changes you could make. Even something as simple as eating one meal each day without a screen can create meaningful space for presence and connection.

Gaze at the sky

Spending time in nature, whenever possible, is a powerful act of self-care. While not everyone has easy access to woodlands, mountains or the sea, we can all take a moment to step outside, breathe in the fresh air and connect with the world beyond our walls.

Try cloud gazing during the day – let your gaze soften and your thoughts drift – or, on clear nights, turn your attention to the stars. Simply looking up at the moon and constellations can offer a sense of perspective and calm. Your ancestors once did this every night – a quiet ritual of wonder, reflection and connection to the cosmos.

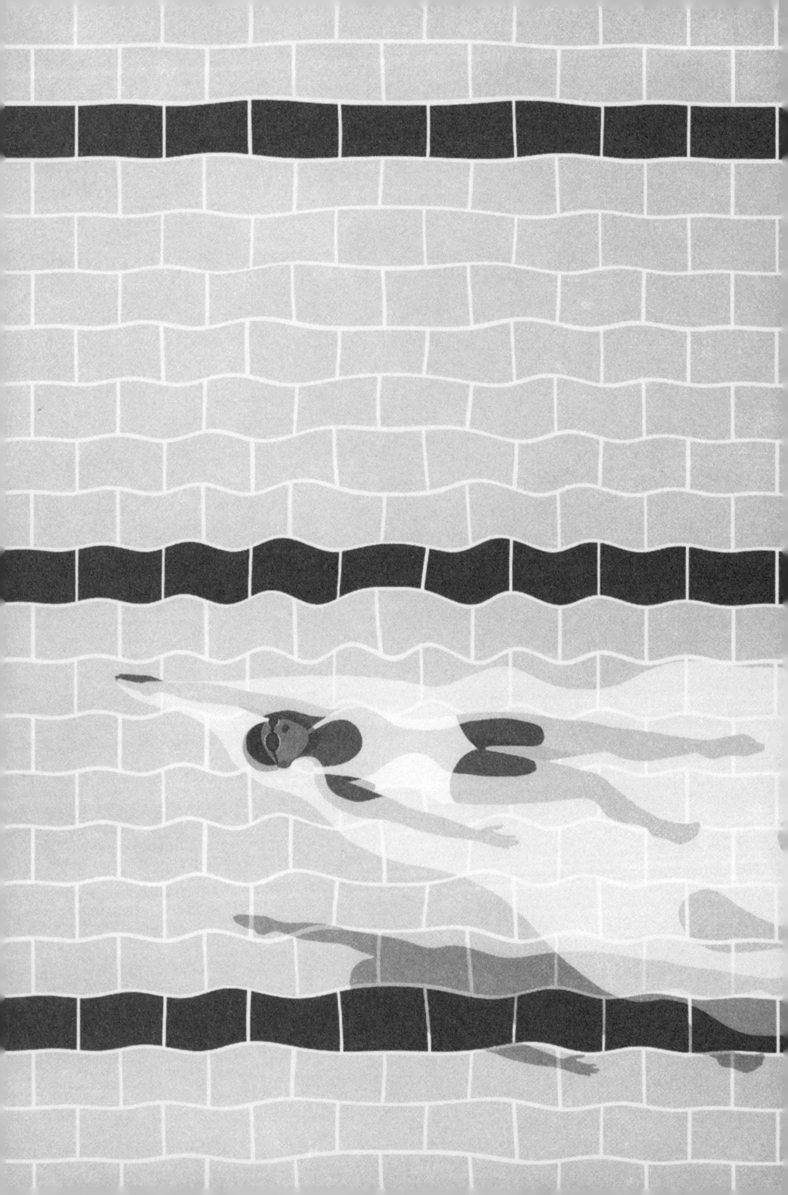

Chapter Four

BELONGING AND BECOMING

True wellbeing emerges in meaningful connection

Nurture relationships

Healthy relationships are among the most enriching parts of life – and nurturing them is a meaningful form of self-care.

One of the simplest and most powerful ways to care for our connections is by being fully present. When spending time with friends or family, practise giving them your full attention – listen deeply, make eye contact and try to avoid using your phone. These small acts of presence can have a big impact.

It might feel vulnerable at first, but expressing appreciation and gratitude strengthens relationships. When you notice qualities you admire in someone, let them know. Heartfelt words can deepen bonds and create lasting connections.

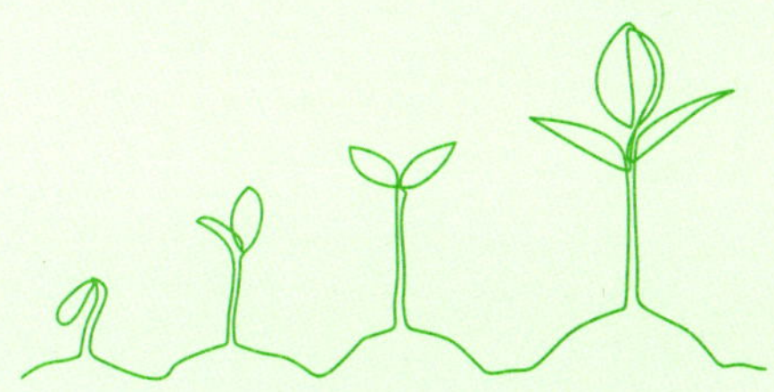

Take time to reflect on the balance in your relationships. Are you giving more than you receive – or are you receiving without giving? If so, how can you bring about more balance and restore harmony?

Finally, prioritize connection in your calendar. Whether it's a weekly phone call with a family member who lives far away, regular family meals or gatherings with friends or your community, relationships thrive when we tend to them with care and intention.

Create boundaries

Boundaries are essential in relationships – not only to protect your energy, but also to create space for genuine connection. While many people find it difficult to set boundaries, often fearing disappointment or conflict, it's important to remember that healthy boundaries can be set with clarity and kindness.

Try these boundary-setting journal exercises:

1. When was the last time I said yes when, truthfully, I wanted to say no?
2. Where in my life do I feel stretched too thin?
3. What does it feel like when one of my boundaries is crossed?
4. What would it be like to honour my needs as much as I honour the needs of others?
5. What's one small boundary I could set right now?

The art of saying "no"

The word "no" is a complete sentence. Yet so often, we feel compelled to justify or apologize for saying it. Setting boundaries is one of the most powerful ways we can care for ourself. Saying "no" allows us to protect our time, energy and emotional wellbeing – creating space for what truly matters.

Whether it's turning down a social invitation, stepping away from overcommitment or simply choosing not to explain ourselves, each "no" we offer can be an art of courage and clarity.

Honouring our limits is not about shutting people out, it's about making room for what nourishes us. When we say "no" with intention, we're also saying "yes" to ourselves.

Here are some gentle yet clear ways to say no:

- "Thank you for thinking of me, but I can't commit to that right now"
- "I'm focusing on other things right now, so I need to pass"
- "That's not something I can do at the moment"
- "I appreciate the invitation, but I need to rest"
- "That doesn't feel fully aligned for me right now"

Every time you say "no" with kindness and without guilt, you are saying "yes" to your deeper needs.

Live with purpose

For all people, feeling a sense of purpose is a vital part of self-care. It doesn't need to be grand or life-changing – often, purpose can be found in simple places.

- Reading bedtime stories to a child every night
- Growing a vegetable or flower garden
- Helping an elderly neighbour with their weekly errands
- Creating art that expresses emotional concepts
- Bringing love and warmth to your everyday interactions

The key to living with purpose is that it feels meaningful to you. Answer the following questions to discover what naturally draws your interest and energy:

1. Which activities make time seem to disappear?
2. What kind of conversations do you find yourself leaning into?
3. What issues spark a sense of compassion or justice within you?
4. What do friends consistently seek your help with?

These questions can help you understand your personal and unique sources of meaning. Remember that purpose evolves through different stages of life.

Connect to something larger

Human beings naturally seek connection to something greater than ourselves – whether that's the land beneath our feet, a creative force, a sense of community, a spiritual tradition or simply the vastness of the universe. One way to connect to something bigger is by noticing what inspires a moment of transcendence in your life.

For example:

- Meditation, prayer or ritual
- The moon and stars
- Music that moves you to tears
- Unexpected kindness from a stranger
- The perfect unfurling of a flower
- Stories of your ancestors and their journeys

Taking time to connect with something greater than yourself can be one of the most powerful self-care practices. It offers a sense of belonging and reminds you that you are part of something vast, interconnected and deeply meaningful.

Discover your self-care values

Personal values are the principles that guide your decisions and give your life a sense of direction. When you understand your core values, self-care becomes more intentional and aligned. Being clear on your core values can help you:

- Make decisions with greater confidence
- Set boundaries to protect what's important to you
- Invest your time and energy wisely
- Find a deeper meaning in everyday actions

This practice begins with awareness. It's the quiet recognition of your needs, your limits and what brings you ease. These values are not rules, but gentle anchors – reminders to care for yourself in ways that feel true to you. On the next page, you'll find a closer look at each of them. Let them meet you where you are and guide you to where you need to go.

Balance
Rest
Boundaries
Authenticity
Compassion
Peace
Growth
Self-respect
Pleasure
Connection

Nature
Creativity
Play
Presence
Nourishment
Simplicity
Wonder
Intuition
Gentleness
Wholeness

Release perfectionism

Perfectionism often begins as an emotional shield – a way to protect ourselves from criticism, judgement or the fear of not being enough. While it can sometimes make us feel safe, it can also hold us back from fully experiencing the messy, beautiful and unpredictable nature of life. On the opposite page is a gentle ritual to help soften the grip of perfectionism and create space for self-acceptance.

1. Safely light a candle in a quiet space.
2. On a piece of paper, note how perfectionism might be holding you back.
3. Hold your paper and speak out loud: "I fully release the need to be perfect."
4. Carefully burn the paper in a safe environment and watch it slowly transform into ash, recognizing the alchemy you are creating.
5. Take a few deep breaths to feel into this act of release.

You can use this releasing ritual whenever negative thought patterns are weighing you down.

Financial self-care

Financial self-care involves nurturing your relationship with money in a compassionate and practical way. Many people find budgeting, saving or managing money challenging – this can often lead to stress.

Top tips to ease financial stress

- Approach your finances with compassion and remember that money blocks are often a reflection of systemic issues – not personal failings
- Take some time to write down the way you feel about money and the emotions it evokes – remember that we all have different starting points, skills and resources

- Set aside some time each week (or at least once a month) to check your finances and stay updated on your outgoings – try to have a clear understanding of what is coming in and what is going out
- If you're looking to make significant changes, start with one small, manageable habit – such as saving a little money each time you get paid, or cancelling a subscription that you no longer use
- Remember that financial wellbeing is about holding a sense of peace and possibility around money

A gratitude meditation

Gratitude is a powerful form of self-care because it shifts our focus from what's missing in our lives to recognizing what is beautifully abundant.

On the following page is a gratitude meditation that offers a simple way to cultivate this perspective, helping you reconnect with yourself and the world around you with greater warmth and clarity.

1. Find a comfortable position and gently close your eyes. Take a few deep breaths.
2. Think of one specific aspect of your life that fills you with appreciation. It can be as simple as love for your pet, being proud of your garden or closeness with a particular person.
3. As you inhale deeply, imagine your breath flowing directly into this aspect of your life, filling it with more and more energy.
4. As you exhale, release any tiredness, frustration or feelings of lack.
5. Do this for 5–10 minutes, then, when you're ready, slowly open your eyes and take a deep breath.

Permission to play

Play is a wonderfully important element of self-care!

As adults, we often forget how to engage in activities purely for joy. Think about the activities that delighted you as a child – whether it was drawing, dancing, climbing trees or making up stories – and explore ways to bring them back into your life.

For example, if you loved making potions from flowers, why not try foraging and then cooking something with what you find?

Hobbies are a fun way to practise self-care because they carve out dedicated space for joy, curiosity and creative play.

Build a creative practice

For many people, creativity is an incredibly effective form of self-care. Engaging in any kind of creative expression – whether big or small – can spark joy, ease stress and help you process emotions in a healthy way. Here are some ideas to get your creative juices flowing:

- Use coloured pencils, markers or paints to express your feelings
- Sketch or write about the natural world around you
- Experiment in the kitchen with flavours and ingredients
- Dance to music that moves you
- Create collages using old magazines, photos and other materials

- Try clay or pottery work – feel the earth between your fingers
- Sing or hum – use your voice to create sounds that you can feel in your body
- Create simple flower arrangements
- Take photographs of small details that capture your eye
- Experiment with simple embroidery, knitting or beading
- Plant seeds and tend to their growth
- Write or record short stories, real or imagined
- Create natural pieces of art from stones, bark, flowers, feathers and leaves

Remember – you don't have to be an accomplished artist to be creative. Anyone can do it!

Slow hope

As you continue on your self-care journey, remember that wellbeing is not a destination, but an ongoing practice. Each small act of care – for yourself, for others and for the world around you – gently weaves together a more whole, grounded and healing way of being.